PTSD

Posttraumatic Stress Disorder

Alternative Resources for Recovery

Suka Chapel-Horst, RN, Ph.D.

PSTSD – Posttraumatic Stress Disorder
Alternative Resources for Recovery

Author: Suka Chapel-Horst, RN, PhD, QMHP, CPLT

Published by:
Brainworks Publishing
638 Spartanburg Highway, Suite #70-175
Hendersonville, NC 28792

www.AriseAlcoholRecovery.com
www.IMRIWellness.org

ISBN: 10-1494319926
ISBN: 13- 978-1494319922

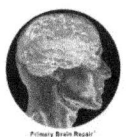

PRIMARY BRAIN REPAIR

Primary Brain Repair focuses on providing the brain, body, and spirit with the basic requirements for health and wellbeing. It's the first line response to all illnesses and disorders. It involves the use of natural micronutrients, nutrition therapy, exercise, and stress relief.

Optimal health can be achieved by most people by following these guidelines. For individuals who need more intensive treatment, these basic health steps will be the foundation that allows advanced treatment to be effective. When primary brain repair is not addressed, medications and counseling have little long-term effect.

At Integrative Memory Research Institute our mission and passion is to educate the public and healthcare professionals about the most advanced methods for obtaining optimal health, naturally. Based on the latest neuroscience and biochemical research, along with years of experience, Dr. Suka offers leading-edge knowledge and how-to information to those who are seeking real recovery versus symptom relief.

Using simple, but effective, recovery tools, *Primary Brain Repair* will improve the health of everyone who applies it. How can that be? Simply, because we go back to the basics of how the brain and body are designed to work. The answer is in nature, and the method is natural.

We are passionate about helping you. That's why we've created self-help books and DVDs to guide you through the process.

www.IMRIWellness.org
417-380-3254

Other books and DVDs by Dr. Suka Chapel-Horst

WORKBOOKS

How to Quit Drinking for Good and Feel Good

"Why Do I Feel This Way?" Natural Healing for Optimal Health and
    Relief from Moods and Depression

BOOKS

Take a Leap of Faith

DVD

Depression – Ten Different Sources / Ten Different Approaches
    Your Guide to Finding and Treating the Real Underlying Cause

BOTTOM LINE BOOKS
BOOKS/DVD PowerPoint Presentations

Wellness Simplified – How Food affects Moods, Bodies, and Behaviors

Say Goodbye to Moods and Depression

The Real Cause and Solution for Alcohol Addiction

The Gift – A Sound Mind for Life

Cannabinoids: Marijuana, THC, CBN, Cannabis, CBD – The Hundredth
    Monkey Cure

Trick or Treat – What Your Doctor isn't Telling You about
    Mood Altering Medications

These books and DVD's can be ordered through:
www.AriseAlcoholRecovery.com
www.IMRIWellness.org or by calling: 417-380-3254

ABOUT THE AUTHOR

Dr. Suka has over forty-five years of experience as a Registered Nurse in the fields of mental health, criminal justice, addictions, and wellness education. She worked in hospitals, addiction and detox centers, residential treatment centers for the mentally ill, residential homes for the mentally challenged, locked facilities and residential treatment homes for teenagers with criminal histories. Dr. Suka has been a jail nurse, home health nurse, operating room nurse, infertility education nurse, and owner of a nursing services business serving residential treatment centers.

In 1984 Dr. Suka completed a seminary program and was ordained as an inter-faith minister. This led to training as a hospital chaplain, and to becoming chaplain to a county sheriff's department. Her doctorate is in the ministry.

Dr. Suka is the founder and director of *ARISE* Alcohol Recovery, LLC, offering an out-patient program and two self-help alcohol recovery programs that can be done in the privacy and comfort of one's home while continuing with normal daily activities or work responsibilities.

She is a wellness consultant and a Certified Past Lives Therapist®, author, and speaker.

INTRODUCTION

Posttraumatic Stress Disorder (PTSD) is a debilitating condition affecting multitudes of individuals and families throughout the world. It creates untold suffering for years and decades after the original trauma occurred.

Traditional treatment consists of counseling and medication. It's clear, however, that these methods of treatment, in large part, have failed to alleviate the condition known as PTSD.

With advances in the fields of neuroscience, biochemistry, bioenergy, and psychology, more resources have become available which have the potential to rescue those suffering from this condition and return them to a normal and healthy life, free from the memories that haunt and debilitate them.

This *Bottom Line Book*, in simple language and format, is an introduction to the underlying biochemical and psychological causes of PTSD, and to some of the advances in science and psychology that are currently helping people recover from this disorder.

I make no claims or promises of recovery from using these practices. Rather, recovery depends upon how committed and dedicated the person with PTSD is to applying the techniques and strategies offered.

If I could give any advice, it would be to remain open to alternatives to traditional medical treatment. What seems unusual and different now may well become the standard of care in the future. Why wait when so much is already available today?

"Dr. Suka" Chapel-Horst
December 2013
Etowah, North Carolina

CONTENTS

1   WHAT IS POSTTRAUMATIC STRESS DISORDER?

Due to severe trauma or a life-threatening event, PTSD can happen to anyone, anytime, anywhere. It can happen to children, teens, and adults. It's an unconscious, automatic, survival reaction to events. PTSD, as it is commonly known, used to be called "shell shock" or "combat stress".

People who have experienced severe trauma or life-threatening events felt like their lives, or the lives of others, were in danger and that they had no control over what was happening. They may have witnessed people being injured or dying and/or been physically harmed themselves.

Factors that can increase the likelihood of a traumatic event leading to PTSD are 1) the intensity and duration of the trauma, 2) being hurt or losing a loved one, 3) being physically close to the traumatic event, 4) feeling that they were not in control, and 5) having a lack of support after the event.

The symptoms of PTSD may not surface for months or years after the event or after returning from deployment in the military. The symptoms may also come and go.

PTSD SYMPTOMS
People with PTSD will be upset by things that remind them of what happened. They may have nightmares, vivid memories, and flashbacks of events. They may feel emotionally cut off from others. They may feel numb or lose interest in things they used to care about. They may become depressed or think that they are always in danger.

They may feel anxious, jittery, or irritated, and experience a sense of panic that something bad is about to happen. They may have difficulty sleeping, have trouble keeping their mind on one thing, and have a hard time relating to or getting along with their spouse, family, or friends.

People with PTSD frequently avoid places or things that remind them of what happened. Constant drinking or use of drugs to numb their feelings is common. They may start working all the time to occupy their mind, or pull away from other people and become isolated. They may act out by harming themselves or others.

Some individuals suffer from PTSD for years without relief. This *Bottom Line Book* offers some alternative resources that can bring relief, once and for all.

PART ONE

UNDERLYING BIOCHEMICAL CAUSE

2 UNDERLYING BIOCHEMICAL CAUSE OF PTSD

MEMORY STORAGE

The outer surface, in the front portion of the brain, is called the NEOCORTEX and it's the part of the brain that thinks, analyzes, and intuits. It's where we foresee the consequences of our actions. It allows us to be aware of and manage our emotions if we choose to do so (and if our brain is biochemically healthy). The language of the neocortex is words and numbers and it's where we have conscious awareness of our emotions.

The LIMBIC SYSTEM, which is in all mammals, lies within the center of the brain. It's a primitive brain consisting of the amygdala, hippocampus, hypothalamus, thalamus, and the pituitary. While all of these areas are very important, to keep it simple, I'll focus on just two of these areas, the amygdala and the hippocampus.

The limbic system is the automatic first responder to all events, the front line defense. Its language is the five senses: seeing, hearing, feeling, tasting, and smelling.

The neocortex, at the top and front of the brain, is always "after the fact" meaning that the limbic system responds first and then thinking takes place. So when we become aware of an event and think about it, it has already happened and our thinking is truly "after the fact".

The limbic system is where memories are processed. Its response is instinctual and its only purpose is to survive. The senses trigger stored memories and, based upon the content of the stored memories, emotions are created. Mad, glad, sad, and scared.

The AMYGDALA is about the size of a walnut and it sits at the head of the hippocampus. It's the main processing area for emotional memories. The amygdala helps the hippocampus sort and store memories, especially ones with emotion. It evaluates the emotional impact that thoughts carry. The more emotion attached to the thoughts, the more likely memories will go into long-term storage.

Panic can cause amnesia. Shock can cause an emotional shutdown, but the images will still go into storage. The physical energy responses associated with the shock, or energy blocks, will be stored in cellular memory, as well.

The word "hippocampus" comes from the Greek language. "Hyppos" means "horse" and "Kampos" means "sea monster". The hippocampus region of the brain looks like a sea horse with the head near the amygdala while the body curves away from the head ending in what looks like a smaller tail.

The HIPPOCAMPUS is the brain's memory center. It stores some short-term and a few long-term memories. It stores dry unemotional facts and ships most long-term memories with emotion to the temporal lobe.

The temporal lobe controls most memory, hearing, and language. Emotional memories are stored in every cell in our body and so they're called "cellular memory". Memories are stored as images, not words or numbers. They cluster with similar images and evoke an emotional response when triggered.

The brain doesn't know the difference between imagined and real events. Recalling a traumatic event will trigger the same physical and emotional stress response that occurred during the initial event.

Recalling or remembering an emotionally traumatic event creates a new memory of the event and adds it to already stored cellular memories increasing its negative emotional power. The physical body then re-enacts the stress response and the emotional charge is, thus, increased. The person is actually being re-traumatized by this recall. That's why traditional talk-therapy can actually embed trauma more deeply into a person's psyche.

Healing requires that the negative energy charge, or physical energy caused by the stress response, be neutralized in order to decrease the traumatic effects of memory recall. In other words, we have to stop the stress response from occurring during recall of the event.

Thoughts and emotions are measurable energy. Traumatic memory recall creates an energy response. Thus, healing requires a transformation or dissipation of the negative energy.

3 THE STRESS RESPONSE

The limbic system, in the center of the brain, is survival oriented. When it feels threatened by what it's sensing and remembering from stored memories, it initiates the stress response.

First, the hormone, adrenaline, is released from the adrenal glands. Adrenaline prepares the physical body for fight or flight. It raises heart rate and increases blood supply to the muscles. It increases blood sugar for more energy and increases blood flow to the brain thus activating cognitive function and memory recording, unless the person is experiencing panic. Severe panic can cause amnesia.

At the same time, cortisol, the primary stress responder, is released. Cortisol releases sugar (glucose) into the blood stream which enhances the brain's activity. It curbs nonessential activities such as digestion, the reproductive system, and growth processes in children. It also alters immune system functioning.

Adrenaline is a short term response lasting just minutes, enough to prepare the physical body for action. Cortisol, however, stays in the system for several hours.

Cortisol is not harmful in moderate amounts. However, when it's produced in excess, day after day, as the result of chronic, unrelenting stress, cortisol is so toxic to the brain that it not only kills and injures brain cells by the billions, but it also destroys the biochemical integrity of the brain. This is the number one factor behind both the aging process and eventual dementia and Alzheimer's.

Chronic cortisol stress response slows down digestion leading to malnutrition. It represses the reproductive system creating poor libido, difficult menses, and infertility, and it retards growth in children. It alters immune system functioning causing illness, chronic fatigue, immune system disorders, and more.

The hippocampus, the brain's memory center, is the first part of brain to be damaged due to chronic stress. Trauma creates a toxic biochemical overload, a brain on fire.

Operating through the neocortex, a biochemically healthy brain can help manage emotions, reactions, memory and memory recall. A compromised brain, biochemically imbalanced, is at the mercy of emotions and fight or flight (survival) reactions.

4 COMMUNICATION SYSTEM
BRAIN CHEMISTRY SIMPLIFIED

It's not important to remember the following details. It is important to be aware that all brain chemicals work together, as well as individually, just as all organs and systems work together. We are holistic beings.

There are approximately 100 billion neurons in the brain. These brain cells are not connected to each other. Information is sent from one neuron to the next by chemicals that carry an electromagnetic charge, or "message". What is important to remember is that these neurotransmitters are proteins and proteins are made up of amino acids.

Let's consider six neurotransmitters that are related to memory.
- Acetylcholine
- Dopamine
- Norepinephrine
- Serotonin
- GABA
- Endorphins

Acetylcholine is the "Superstar" neurotransmitter of memory and thought. It's the most abundant neurotransmitter in the brain and is highly concentrated in the hippocampus, the memory center. It triggers muscle action and concentration.

Symptoms of an acetylcholine <u>deficiency</u> are:
- Subdued or depressed mood
- Anxiety
- Inability to experience pleasure

- Difficulty concentrating
- Mental fatigue
- Mental confusion
- Memory problems
- Decreased motivation
- Feeling overly sleepy
- Fretfulness
- Irritability or anger
- Sadness, tearfulness
- Introversion
- Paranoia
- Feel taken advantage of
- Difficulty understanding or performing tasks
- Pessimistic, negative ideation or rumination
- Feelings of helplessness and hopelessness
- Difficulty with complex thought processes
- More and vivid dreaming & higher incidence of nightmares

Dopamine is the "Energizer Bunny" neurotransmitter. It's a "feel good" chemical that stimulates, excites, and motivates us. It helps us to concentrate and take action. **Dopamine is the brain's natural cocaine.**

Symptoms of a dopamine <u>deficiency</u> are:
- Reduced ability to feel pleasure
- Flat, bored, apathetic and low enthusiasm
- Depressed
- Low drive and motivation
- Procrastination
- Difficulty concentrating
- Slowed thinking
- Poor memory
- Low energy
- Unmotivated
- Shy/introverted
- Low libido or impotence
- Sleep too much
- Trouble getting out of bed
- Put on weight easily
- Mentally and physically fatigued easily

Before going on, let me clarify a word that I'll be using as it relates to biochemistry. A "precursor" is a compound that participates in a chemical reaction that produces another compound, for example, hydrogen and oxygen are "precursors" to water. Dopamine is a precursor to norepinephrine which I'll be talking about next.

Norepinephrine is the "Bright" neurotransmitter as well as a hormone. It elevates our mood and excites us. It carries memories from short-term to long-term storage. It helps regulate the sex drive and stimulates the metabolic rate. **Norepinephrine is the brain's natural amphetamine.**

Symptoms of a norepinephrine <u>excess</u> are:
- Prevention of memories
- Interferes with rational thought and decision making
- Insomnia
- Decreases sex drive
- Kills appetite
  (Diet pills stimulate the production of norepinephrine)

Symptoms of a norepinephrine <u>deficiency</u> are:
- Diminished energy, interest and motivation
- Depression
- Decreased sense of awareness
- Constant feelings of hunger
- Low energy levels
- Chronic fatigue
- Decreased mental focus
- Variations of Attention Deficit Disorder
- Lack of motivation
- Poor problem solving

Serotonin is the brain's "Sunshine" neurotransmitter. It relaxes us, affects our moods, sleep, appetite, and our perception. **Serotonin is the brain's natural antidepressant.**

Serotonin regulates both dopamine and norepinephrine levels.

Symptoms of a serotonin <u>deficiency</u> are:
- Depression
- Anxiety
- Irritability
- Impatience
- Impulsiveness
- Inability to concentrate
- Weight gain or unexplained weight loss
- Overeating and/or carbohydrate cravings
- Poor dream recall
- Insomnia

Both low serotonin and low dopamine levels lead to depression.

GABA is the brain's "Chill Out" neurotransmitter. It's a sedative and it reduces anxiety. **GABA is the brain's natural Valium.**

GABA assists serotonin in managing dopamine and nor-epinephrine levels. Normal GABA and low serotonin and/or low dopamine lead to depression. Low GABA and low serotonin and/or low dopamine lead to depression with anxiety.

Symptoms of a GABA <u>deficiency</u> are:
- Difficulty relaxing
- Easily stressed or overwhelmed
- Overworked or pressured
- Body uptight or stiff
- Sometimes feel weak or shaky
- Increased stress if skip a meal
- Bothered by loud noises, lights, too much activity

Endorphins are the "Love Bug" neurotransmitters. The endorphins are a group of chemicals that act *like* a neurotransmitter. They provide comfort and pleasure. They are the **brain's natural pain killers (opiates)** for both emotional and physical pain.

Symptoms of an endorphin <u>deficiency</u> are:
- Discomfort
- Persistent pain – Emotional & Physical
- Stress and frustration
- Low interest, focus, concentration

The response to these deficiencies is to crave caffeine, colas, sugar, and bad carbohydrates. People will abuse alcohol, marijuana, opiates, and nicotine or depend upon antidepressants & benzodiazepines.

Why? ...because these substances work. They stimulate the release of neurotransmitters, but only...*temporarily* and they all create dependence or an addiction to them.

Mood altering medications (antidepressants, benzodiazepines, antipsychotics) work on the same principle as does alcohol, marijuana, cocaine, nicotine, heroin, sugar, and junk food. Over time, the conditions become chronic, not better, with prolonged use.

All these substances manipulate brain chemistry to make us feel better or to reduce unwanted symptoms. However, there is a down side to using these substances over long periods of time.

I've written a little book called *Trick or Treat. What Your Doctor isn't Telling You about Mood Altering Medications.* If you are considering taking any of these medications, or are already on them, and want to understand how they affect the brain, and ultimately your health, you'll want to read this book. (See the Appendix.)

If an individual had imbalanced brain chemistry *before* the traumatic event occurred, there is a greater chance that PTSD will result. Those with balanced brain chemistry will have more internal physiological resources to deal with severe trauma which may be why some people develop PTSD and others don't, even though they share the same or similar experiences.

5 REBALANCE BRAIN AND BODY CHEMISTRY

I'm going to give you several resources to assist with recovery from PTSD.

AMINO ACIDS

To begin let's look at the magic of amino acids. All living things are made of protein. Amino acids are the building blocks of protein and neurotransmitters are made of amino acids. Only amino acids and their co-factors can restore neurotransmitter levels to normal. Medications *manipulate* brain chemistry. Amino acids *restore* brain chemistry.

Precursors are substances from which another substance is formed, especially by metabolic reaction.

Some Natural Precursors to the Neurotransmitters
- Lecithin has lots of choline in it which is a precursor to **acetylcholine**.
- Amino acids L-Tyrosine and L-Phenylalanine are precursors to **Dopamine**.
- Amino acid Tryptophan becomes 5HTP which is a precursor to **Serotonin** and **Melatonin.**
- Amino acids L-Glutamine and GABA are precursors to the **GABA** neurotransmitter.
- The vitamin B called Inositol is a precursor to **GABA**.
- DL-Phenylalanine is a precursor to the **Endorphins, Dopamine,** and **Norepinephrine**

Imbalanced brain chemistry can be normalized with specific formulas of amino acids combined with their specific co-factors (vitamins, minerals, essential fatty acids, enzymes, trace elements). These co-factors are necessary for the amino acids to metabolize properly. Mood and mind altering medications manipulate brain chemistry but also deplete the neurotransmitters over time. Amino acids and their co-factors rebuild the neurotransmitters and do it naturally.

To aid you in restoring brain chemistry with amino acids, I've written a book called *"Why Do I Feel This Way?" – Natural Healing for Optimal Health and Relief from Moods and Depression.* This book contains a Mood Meter and written tests to help you discover what neurotransmitters you may be low in, if any. The written tests are very accurate because they are based on the specific symptoms that are caused by specific neurotransmitter deficiencies.

The book also contains amino acid protocols - the what, when, and how to use amino acids. Please be aware that people should not just go out and buy amino acids. While they have no side effects when taken **appropriately**, some amino acids should **not** be taken under certain conditions or if a person is on some specific medications. If a person doesn't need an amino acid and takes it, she may have a short-term (minutes) negative reaction. That's why the book also contains a complete "**precautions**" list to check out before taking the amino acids. This book is a self-help, how-to manual, easy to read and understand.

When purchasing amino acids and food supplements, always choose quality over cost. Inexpensive amino acids and other supplements are sometimes made in China. These products are cheap because Chinese products have no quality control, no supervision, and no oversight. Even worse, many of these products have been found to have little or no amino acids, vitamins, or herbs in them at all.

NEURONUTRIENTS – CO-FACTORS

Amino acids can't work alone. In order for them to be metabolized, co-factors - vitamins, minerals, enzymes, essential fatty acids, and trace elements - are required.

For example, let's look at just the vitamin B's. When there is a deficiency in these nutrients, multiple symptoms may develop such as:

Emotional Symptoms due to a Vitamin B Deficiency

- Confusion
- Poor concentration
- Poor memory
- Depression
- Insomnia
- Anxiety
- Hyperactivity
- Agitation
- Impulsive
- Anger
- Irritability
- Quarrelsome
- Mood swings
- Panic attacks
- Obsessive-compulsive

Physical Symptoms due to a Vitamin B Deficiency

- Hyperactivity
- Headache
- Fatigue
- Insomnia
- Convulsions
- Agitation
- Decreased sex drive
- Tension
- Dizziness
- Gastric ulcers
- High blood pressure
- High cholesterol

- Arteriosclerosis
- Constipation
- Hair loss
- Skin eruptions
- Kidney /Liver impairment
- Extreme nervous exhaustion

SUGAR

Sugar, in all its forms, is the number one addiction of most Americans. It is FOUR times more addictive than cocaine. Excess sugar is a drug that POISONS the body and life.

List of Some Sugar Names

Agave nectar	Evaporated	Lactose
Barbados sugar	cane juice	Malt syrup
Barley malt	Ethyl maltol	Maltodextrin
Beet sugar	Florida Chrystals	Maltose
Blackstrap molasses	Free Flowing	Mannitol
Brown sugar	Fructose	Artificial maple syrup
Buttered syrup	Fruit juice	Molasses
Cane crystals	Fruit juice	Muscovado sugar
Cane juice crystals	concentrate	Organic raw sugar
Cane sugar	Galactose	Panocha
Caramel	Glucose	Powdered sugar
Carob syrup	Glucose solids	Raw sugar
Castor sugar	Golden sugar	Refiner's syrup
Confectioner's sugar	Golden syrup	Rice syrup
Corn syrup	Granulated sugar	Sorbitol
Corn sweetener	Grape sugar	Sorghum syrup
Corn syrup solids	Grape juice	Splenda
Crystalline fructose	concentrate	Sucrose
Date sugar	HFCS	Sugar
Demerara sugar	High-fructose	Syrup
Dextrin	corn syrup	Table sugar
Dextran	Honey	Treacle
Dextrose	Icing sugar	Turbinado sugar
Diastatic malt	Invert sugar	Yellow sugar
Diatase mannose		

To be PTSD free means healing the body, mind, and spirit. Choices have to be made. What is the goal? How much is freedom from suffering worth? We can't blame outer circumstances for our problems if we're not willing to do what it takes to have good health. We can make a huge, huge start by largely cutting down or giving up the poison of sugar.

All Whites are Sugar

- Ice cream
- Pasta
- White bread
- Pizza crust
- White rice
- White potatoes
- White flour baked goods

Our personal physician told my husband recently that if all of his patients gave up sugar, he would lose 70% of them. That's a powerful statement.

Hypoglycemia, or low blood sugar, occurs when we eat lots of sugar, in any form, on a regular basis. Too much insulin is released to metabolize the sugar. When all the sugar is metabolized, the result is excess insulin and low blood sugar. That's the condition called hypoglycemia.

Symptoms of Hypoglycemia (Low Blood Sugar) are:

- Unprovoked anxieties
- Exhaustion
- Mental confusion
- Forgetfulness
- Irritability
- Insomnia
- Constant worrying
- Internal trembling
- DEPRESSION
- ANGRY OUTBURSTS
- VIOLENCE
- SUICIDE

Note that there can be serious repercussions from low blood sugar.

The Standard American Diet (SAD) is junk food. Americans have the poorest nutritional standard in the world and the most malnutrition. For too many families, fast foods and junk foods are the family's only meals. We see the results in the increase of childhood disorders, obesity, heart problems, diabetes, cancer, and ultimately in dementia and Alzheimer's. Learning problems, behavioral problems, and violence have increased with the over-consumption of these non-foods.

Why do we put on unwanted weight? People will eat junk food, drink colas and then try to avoid eating fats! Check out the "fat myth".

Fat doesn't make us fat. Sugar makes us fat. Our bodies need healthy fat. Eat real butter, drink 100% fat milk unless allergic to dairy. If allergic to dairy, drink almond milk, and cook with butter or coconut oil (if not allergic to dairy).

HEALTHY NUTRITION

Farms aren't what they used to be. There is very little healthy nutrition in foods today because the soil is so depleted of nutrients. Failure to rotate crops depletes the bacteria that feed nutrients to the plants. This is another reason why we need to regularly consume food supplements.

Foods to avoid are:
- Hydrogenated fats
- Cooking oils
- Processed and canned foods
- White bread
- Chips and cookies
- Lunch meats
- Fruit juices

Babies are being given fruit juices that are almost wholly sugar. They are addicted to sugar before the age of two. Why are we surprised at the rapidly climbing childhood obesity rate and increased behavioral problems, including bullying? Sugar = AD(H)D.

Eat three wholesome meals daily. Avoid GMO's (Genetically Modified Organisms). Many health issues are the result of eating these foods, including asthma, autism, and infertility, to name just a few.

GMO Foods
- Corn
- Soy
- Cottonseed
- Canola oil
- Sugar beets
- Hawaiian papaya
- Some zucchini
- Some squash

Many victims of PTSD are suffering from allergies. Wheat and dairy products are the most common. Name a symptom and it can be the result of allergies, including some very severe symptoms. Convicted criminals often drink twice as much milk as the general population. In fact, some of their violent behavior can be directly attributed to milk allergies. Surprised? (Much more of this information can be found in the book *"Why Do I Feel This Way?" – Natural Healing for Optimal Health and Relief from Moods and Depression.* See the Appendix.)

Water
Drink six to eight glasses of water every day. Our bodies are about 70% water. When the level is too low we can experience stress related symptoms.

Homeopathic and naturopathic remedies are natural and holistic products that can assist in recovery. Contact a qualified practitioner for assistance. Don't attempt to be your own doctor. Avoid a "little dab of this and a little dab of that". We are holistic in nature. Knowing how to put all the pieces together, like a picture puzzle, requires knowledge of the picture we want to create.

6 PYROLURIA, TOXIC METALS, ALCOHOL

PYROLURIA

Pyroluria is a stress disorder that's often triggered by severe emotional or physical trauma (think PTSD). Pyrroles are a harmless metabolic byproduct that attaches to zinc and B6, flushing them from the body through the urine.

If someone has about 50% of these symptoms, he or she may have pyroluria, which can be easily treated.

- Depression
- Severe emotional mood swings
- Rages – Poor anger control
- Poor short term memory
- Intolerance of emotional stress
- Intolerance of physical stress
- Absence of dream recall
- Inner tension
- Reading disorders
- Fearful, pessimistic, loners
- Rapid cycling mood swings many times daily
- Morning nausea; no morning appetite
- Sensitivity to bright lights, loud noises, touch
- Frequent infections
- Abnormal fat distribution

These people may appear to be extremely mentally ill and can be very difficult to cope with. They're usually treated with antidepressants, benzodiazepines, and mind altering drugs, and they don't improve because they haven't been tested for pyroluria and they're getting the wrong treatment.

Natural relief of pyroluria is to normalize zinc and B6 levels using multiple supplements. There will be clear improvement in just days and a full effect in just 4 to 6 weeks. (As an aside, pyroluria is the cause of most post-partum depression which can be quickly relieved with the proper treatment.)

Relieving pyroluria won't necessarily cure PTSD. But it will remove the debilitating symptoms that are caused by the zinc/B6 imbalance. If one has pyroluria, very little else in the way of medications or therapy will be effective until it is relieved.

(See the Appendix for laboratory testing without a prescription. **Direct Health: www.pyroluriatesting.com** is the best source. When ordering this test, also request a doctor's consultation for guidance on treatment. Do not attempt to recover from pyroluria by yourself.)

TOXIC METALS

Toxic poisoning can be due to overloads of lead, mercury, arsenic, and cadmium, plus other metals. Veterans, especially, have been exposed to high levels of toxic metals. If one doesn't respond to other methods of treatment, toxic metal testing should be considered.

Toxic symptoms are:
- Depression arising suddenly during a period of relative calm and wellness
- Abdominal pain and cramping
- Increased irritability
- Headaches
- Muscle weakness
- Low energy
- Failure to respond to counseling or psychiatric medications

Cadmium, found in cigarette paper, is especially dangerous. It collects in the kidneys causing permanent damage. Smoking 1 to 2 packs daily can double blood and tissue levels of the metal.

Some military personnel are exposed to high levels of lead in ammunition. Other sources are shallow wells, fertilizers, metal welding, brazing, fireworks, artist's paints, mining operations, industrial plants, paint, and shellfish.

Toxic poisoning may be difficult to diagnose due to low blood levels of the toxin. With treatment there may be a mild worsening the first 10 days as the toxins are removed from the body, followed by steady improvement in the next four to six months. The half-life of lead in the bones is 22 years, so toxic symptoms from lead can last a long time. (See the Appendix for testing laboratories which do not require a prescription.)

ALCOHOL USE

All too often individuals with unresolved PTSD will resort to substance abuse in order to alleviate the symptoms. Alcohol addiction can be a common co-occurring problem. All of the resources I've mentioned in this book are solutions for both alcohol abuse and addiction, as well as PTSD.

However, specific treatment is necessary to rebalance dysfunctional brain chemistry due to alcohol abuse. (See the Bottom Line Book *The Real Cause and Solution for Alcohol Addiction* and the workbook *How to Quit Drinking for Good and Feel Good* in the Appendix section of this book.)

7 ENERGY BLOCKS

It's not enough to improve brain and body chemistry. We still have to eliminate the energy charge, or stress reactions that occur with each memory recall. Conversely, attempting to do energy work without restoring brain chemistry won't work either. And, finally, therapy to uncover and resolve unconscious source trauma gets to the root of everything.

Exercise / Walking

It should come as no surprise that exercise has to be a part of recovery. However, I know that many people don't like to exercise. For those who do, fine. For those who don't, at least thirty minutes of brisk walking every day, or forty minutes every two days, will do it as long as you keep the heart rate up. Breaking a little sweat is a good sign that you're getting a decent workout. Just remember that this is a necessary recovery step.

Body Work

There are many excellent forms of body work that I recommend. They include:

- Massage
- Reflexology
- Acupuncture
- Chiropractic
- Cranial Sacral therapy
- Myofascial Trigger Point therapy

All of these therapies help to release both toxins and stress from the body. They are excellent adjuncts to emotional energy releasing work.

Another very valuable and enjoyable healing method is to regularly get an infra-red dry-heat sauna, as frequently as several times weekly. Saunas release toxins while relaxing muscles. Avoid steam saunas as the temperature can be too hot for a body already under stress.

Many people have acquired heavy amounts of toxic chemicals and these saunas are a great way to release them. Following the sauna, shower down with soap and water to remove the toxins from the skin so that they aren't reabsorbed.

Breathing for stress relief is a most beneficial and immediate resource. Proper breathing can change anxiety into peace in minutes. It can transform fear into relaxation. It can enhance concentration and focus. It releases those neurotransmitters that chill us out, relax us, and bring us comfort.

Taking full deep breaths, breathing deeply into our lungs, allowing the abdomen to expand with the inhalation, relaxes the mind and body. The phrase "take ten" doesn't mean to take ten minutes for a cigarette and coffee break, although some folks think it does. It means to take ten deep and slow breaths to release stress and restore biochemical balance. It's free and can be done anytime, anywhere.

Several healing breath techniques are given in the self-help manual I mentioned before. (*Natural Healing for Optimal Health and Relief from Moods and Depression.*)

Yoga, Tai Chi, and Qigong are wonderful posture and movement methods that have, for centuries, brought stress relief and healing to thousands. There are teachers and classes almost everywhere because Americans are rapidly embracing these ancient practices. You can attend classes or purchase DVDs and follow along at home.

Drumming   Now, who would have thought of drumming as a stress reducing resource? Well, some veterans at Walter Reed Hospital with PTSD are finding that drumming helps them stay calm and focused. Drumming reduces their stress levels and helps to clear out the energy blocks associated with their traumatic memories.

Drumming circles, or just drumming by oneself, has a powerful effect on the heart and all body systems. It brings everything into balance while creating a mesmerizing healing effect.

Drums come in every size, shape, and sound. Try out different ones until you come upon one that "calls" to you. Make drumming part of your daily routine. Every part of your body will respond favorably to it. Additionally, drumming can be a bonding activity for the whole family.

Energy Therapies
Some hands-on or hands-above-the-body energy systems include **Reike, Quantum Touch, Polarity Therapy,** and **Therapeutic Touch.**

These, and other similar methods, can do everything from relaxing a person to outright healing. These methods come to us from centuries of practice. They are able to concentrate and focus energy to specific parts of the body to remove energy blocks and tension.

I know that some of these methods may seem too "far-out" or "weird" to some people. However, these methods are not new. They are tried and true healing methods that are now being more understood through the advent of quantum physics which is explaining the underlying process of how these healing methods work.

Brainwave Technologies
You might explore the growing research and applications of brainwave technologies. They avoid re-traumatization even as they remove the energy blocks connected with traumatic memories. There are several technologies available and more are rapidly being developed.

I have personally experienced twelve hours of brain wave technology. It was quite soothing and relaxing and didn't require any memory recall at all. I only had to observe my brain waves on the computer screen. My brain did all the work outside of my conscious awareness.

Almost every treatment center now uses some form of these technologies. They are rapidly becoming the standard of treatment.

PART TWO

UNDERLYING PSYCHOLOGICAL CAUSE

8 UNDERLYING PSYCHOLOGICAL CAUSE OF PTSD

Present day physical, emotional, and mental pain, and suffering, are the result of unresolved traumatic experiences from our past. The unresolved trauma might be relatively small and insignificant, with minor ongoing effects or it can be extremely debilitating with long lasting outward effects, or anywhere in between.

Nevertheless, the lack of resolution causes ongoing, or chronic internal stress that affects our reactions and behavior toward ourselves and others. It affects how we respond to situations that trigger the known or often hidden memory. I call it, *posttraumatic* stress, and we all experience it to varying degrees. The internal, unresolved memories, even if forgotten, affect our brain and body chemistry. If unconscious, chronic stress continues, without resolution, it eventually leads to unhealthy emotional and mental reactions, and eventually to physical illness and disease.

For example, if we haven't worked through stressful experiences such as being fired, or from causing hurt to another, or feeling betrayed by a trusted friend, or from the loss of a loved one, we are experiencing posttraumatic stress. A mother may grieve over the loss of a child for years without resolving her pain. This can lead to irritability, anger, depression, insomnia, isolation, divorce, gastric and intestinal disorders, or cancer. This is an example of the effects of posttraumatic stress, due to a failure to resolve the hurt and move forward.

Posttraumatic stress *disorder* (PTSD) is a higher degree of reactions due to unresolved, remembered experiences of severe trauma. Reactions include memories and nightmares, flashbacks, avoidance of things related to the event, severe anxiety, sleeplessness, aggressive behavior and angry outbursts which can strike at any time, most commonly when he or she is reminded of the events in question.

The symptoms of unresolved, conscious and unconscious memories of pain and trauma are one of the causes of alcohol addiction. Alcohol abuse and addiction are frequently co-diagnosed with PTSD. Alcohol, mood and mind altering pharmaceutical medications, and illegal drugs, serve to cover up or alleviate unwanted symptoms and memories, at least temporarily. Recovery from alcohol abuse or addiction is the same as for PTSD. (See the Bottom Line Book *The Real Cause and Solution for Alcohol Addiction* in the appendix.)

Unresolved traumatic events may have occurred weeks, months, or years ago. These unresolved memories also include all that we saw, heard, and felt during the first seven years of our life, and while we were in the womb. Yes, we recorded the feelings, thoughts, and words mother experienced during the time we were a tiny fetus in her womb. We simply recorded these in our unconscious mind.

These experiences, from our mother in the womb, and from the first seven years of our life, became our history and our truths because we didn't yet have a conscious mind to discriminate. The stories dictated beliefs to us about how to live in the world, even though the beliefs may have been wrong or harmful.

Sometimes these memories or "stories" may appear to be past life trauma stories that are seeking resolution. It makes no difference whether the stories are fantasy or real, if they happened to us or to mother, or to someone else. If they are in *our* unconscious mind, they become *our* stories, and we will live out the lessons we learned from those stories, even if the lessons are not in our own best interest as we go through life.

When *traumatic* stories in the conscious and unconscious mind are left unresolved, they create unhealthy survival patterns which lead to suffering in our present day life. Those survival patterns, which initially occurred at the time of the earlier trauma, are repeated in our present life when we have similar experiences. Because we haven't resolved the earlier traumatic experience, we continue to re-enact our responses to it in the present.

Emotionally, these survival patterns can show up as anxiety, worry, depression, withdrawal, avoidance, PTSD, addictions, overworking, over exercising, competitiveness, anger, fighting, or violence, for example.

Mentally, these survival patterns can create a victim mentality blaming others, stubbornness, self-righteousness, or superiority, to give just a few examples.

Physically, survival patterns can be the cause of anorexia, diabetes, frequent accidents, digestive disorders, or cancer, for example. In fact, every illness and every disorder is the result of both conscious and unconscious unresolved prior trauma.

So, let's look at what can be done to resolve these underlying psychological causes.

9 SOLUTIONS FOR THE SOUL

Integrative Memory Therapy®

This advanced methodology gets to the originating source of present day issues, allowing for healing and transformation. Unlike other medical and alternative modalities, this process resolves the root of the problem, the unconscious memories of trauma that are controlling present day reactions and behaviors. Healing in the present takes place because the underlying cause is no longer driving behaviors.

Integrative Memory Therapy® is not regression, nor is it hypnosis. Clients are fully conscious at all times. The therapist guides clients to completely resolve their own source trauma. The result is a transformed life in the present.

This therapy is not appropriate for everyone. Clients must be free from mind and mood altering medications that reduce normal emotional responses. (To read testimonials and learn more about *Integrative Memory Therapy®* go to www.IMRIWellness.org or contact Dr. Suka at 417-890-3254.)

Meditation

This is a helpful way to temporarily reverse the stress response. There are many, many ways to meditate and hundreds of books on the subject. All are beneficial. Just find the method that resonates with you. And of course, focusing on the breathing is a meditation technique, as well.

Meridian Tapping

Meridian Tapping is also known as EFT or Emotional Freedom Technique. Energy blockages are released by tapping on energy points on the head and upper body while recalling traumatic events. The emotional charge, or energy block, dissolves leaving the person able to remember the event without negative reactions or uncomfortable emotions, however it does not resolve underlying unconscious memories that are the originating source of PTSD.

This method is now being used with some veterans with PTSD. A DVD can be ordered called *OPERATION: EMOTIONAL FREEDOM   The Answer* from www.operation-emotionalfreedom.com. The book *Meridian Tapping* by Patricia Carrington is an excellent resource for learning meridian tapping.

Belief Management

Life follows thought. What we see, hear, and feel in our imagination becomes our reality in the physical. Fear manifests that which we fear. I recommend the book *Excuses BeGone* by Dr. Wayne Dyer. It comes in both book and CD format.

It's important to learn how to be mindful of our thoughts. Listening to what we are thinking, and observing our behaviors and reactions, is the first step to taking charge of our life. Instead of reacting, we can become the actors, choosing what is best for us in the moment.

While belief management is an important aid to recovery, it should be used in conjunction with other therapies, not as a stand-alone modality.

Spiritual Resources

Whatever makes your heart sing, feels loving and supportive, uplifts you to be more than you could be on your own, is spiritual. Some important qualities to look for are these:

- Gentleness
- Compassion
- Loving
- Positive
- Supportive
- Uplifting
- Helpful
- Hopeful
- Encouraging
- Always available

When you find a place, a center, a church, a group, or a friend who offers you these qualities, you have found a spiritual home. Savor it. If these qualities are not present, move on. Seek elsewhere.

Offer yourself to others in support. You have something to give and in giving, you will receive.

Support and Pets

When I was in my early twenties, my father told me that if we have three good friends in our entire life, we have been fortunate. Sometimes we think that having large numbers of friends means we're a good pal. But friends and good close friends are different.

It only takes one or two to be there for us when we need a friend. And being a friend means we are there for that person, as well. Getting close to another person, revealing one's innermost self is difficult for a person with PTSD. Make the effort.

Pets can be loyal and safe friends. They love unconditionally, if treated with love, and make few demands. These loving pets have the ability to assist in our healing, as well.

Recovery

All of these excellent resources work in conjunction with a biochemically healthy brain and an energetically balanced body. And that is why rebuilding brain chemistry with the proper nutrients and healthy nutrition, along with energy balancing techniques, and psychological healing are all necessary components of a holistic approach to recovery from PTSD.

10 SUMMARY

This, then, is a summary of what we've covered. Many suggestions have been made. Please remember that both brain chemistry and energy blockages have to be addressed, along with resolving the underlying traumatic sources for full recovery. Here's a reminder.

Alternative Resources for Recovery
- Amino acids
- Supplements/Co-factors
- Healthy Nutrition
- Physical Exercise / Walking
- Body Work – Saunas, Massage, etc.
- Breathing
- Meditation
- Energy Medicine
- Belief Management
- Integrative Memory Therapy®
- Spiritual Resources
- Support and Pets

Thank you for reading this *Bottom Line Book*. Please share this information with others and help to save someone's life. It's never too late.

Dr. Suka

December 2013, February 2016
Etowah, North Carolina

RESOURCES

LABORATORY TESTING

SOME RECOMMENDED TESTS
- DHEA and Cortisol Levels
- Thyroid: TSH, Free T3, Free T4
- Neurotransmitter Levels
- Nutrient Evaluation
- Allergies
- Hormone Levels
- Pyroluria
- Toxic Metals (Hair and blood analysis)

SUGGESTED LABORTORIES

Direct Health: www.pyroluriatesting.com
Tests can be ordered directly by the individual on line, through a healthcare provider, or through Dr. Suka. Insurance may cover these tests.

Sanesco Health: www.sanescohealth.com
Sanesco Health offers testing for neurotransmitters and adrenal insufficiency (DHEA and Cortisol). Tests can be ordered through a healthcare provider or through Dr. Suka. Insurance coverage is available.

NeuroScience: www.neurorelief.com
NeuroScience offers neurotransmitter testing. Tests can be ordered through a healthcare provider. Insurance coverage may be available.

Genova Diagnostics: www.gdx.net
Tests can be ordered through a healthcare provider. Insurance coverage may be available.

Life Extension: www.lef.org
Life Extension offers a large variety of tests available to the public without a prescription.

Vitamin D Council: www.vitamindcouncil.com
Inexpensive and accurate Vitamin D testing. No prescription necessary.

TO ORDER HIGH QUALITY SUPPLEMENTS LISTED IN THIS BOOK, CALL ANOVA HEALTH AT 864-408-8320.

Food supplements listed in all of our books can be purchased through Anova Health, also providing WHOLE FOOD supplements. Request a catalog.

Simply call Anova Health and give them the CODE. **Drsuka5** Your order will be shipped the same day, no delays. You will automatically receive a **5% discount and free shipping,** saving you the extra cost of buying supplements of the very best quality. To get these benefits, you must call in your order.

All supplements are of the highest quality available and are suitable for vegetarians. They are free of wheat gluten, soy, milk/dairy, corn, sodium, sugar, starch, artificial coloring, preservatives, and flavoring. I highly recommend the following supplements available through Anova Health.

Amino Acids: All of the amino acids that are listed in my two "how-to" manuals and other books can be ordered through Anova Health. Of course, they can be purchased in many other places, but for the highest quality and purest products, I recommend Anova Health. You may pay a little more, but you will use less and get better results with high quality products.

AvinoCort for managing elevated Cortisol levels caused by chronic stress. Lowering one's cortisol level slows down the aging process and helps to prevent dementia and Alzheimer's. Why use this product? This is a very advanced, stem cell product. Ask the folks at Anova Health for more information if you like. I highly recommend this product for reducing the effects of chronic stress.

Inositol Powder is a normal vitamin B. It is a precursor to GABA, the brain's natural Valium. If you have anxiety, worries, even panic attacks, your inositol level is probably too low. Taking 1000 mg up to four times daily can improve relaxation and reduce anxiety, naturally.

CaliQuil - California Poppy 500 mg Capsules Restores Rest. Prevails over pain. Traditional analgesic and sleep aid. This amazing product really works. Take it before bedtime and see the results. (Does not produce opium, physical dependence, or addiction.)

Acute Pain Relief, a King Bio homeopathic cream, gives excellent relief from joint pain.

Call 864-408-8320 to order these and other products from Anova Health. (If you order on-line, you won't get the discount or free shipping.)

Use the code **drsuka5** to order.

OTHER SUGGESTED RESOURCES FOR QUALITY SUPPLEMENTS
Call and request free catalogs. Order by telephone or on-line.

Life Extension: www.lef.org 1-800-678-8989

Bronson Vitamins: www.bronsonvitamins.com 1-800-235-3200

Cayenne Company: www.cayennecompany.com 1-800-229-3663

For highest quality amino acids call: Dr. Suka at 417-380-3254 or 417-894-8501

ARISE ALCOHOL RECOVERY, LLC PROGRAMS
Director: Suka Chapel-Horst, RN, PhD

Two Self-Help Recovery Programs that can take place in the comfort and privacy of one's home. These programs are based on biochemical restoration of the brain with micronutrient and nutrition therapy using the workbook *How to Quit Drinking for Good and Feel Good.*

- **Self-Managed Program** - Do it on your own following guidelines in the workbook.

- **Managed Program** which includes telephone consultations with Dr. Suka.

Out-Patient Program: This program is based on biochemical restoration of the brain with micronutrient and nutrition therapy using the workbook *How to Quit Drinking for Good and Feel Good.* The out-patient program also includes approximately ten to fifteen sessions of *Integrative Memory Therapy*®.

For more information and testimonials, go to:
www.AriseAlcoholRecovery.com

BOOK (234 pages)
Take a Leap of Faith
Wellness Simplified
by Suka Chapel-Horst, RN, PhD, QMHP, CPLT

If your emotional, mental, or physical health isn't what you wish it to be, you'll find practical suggestions for regaining or maintaining optimal health in this remarkable book. The topics include:

- Halt Premature Aging Now
- Want More Sunshine in Your Life?
- The Cookie Monster - Hypoglycemia
- Five Simple Steps to Optimal Health
- Enjoy Life More
- Your Body Type: Seven Dwarfs and Superman
- Fear versus Love
- Relief from Depression
- Stretching to Wellness
- Bodyguards Got You Covered?
- Bodyguard Banquet
- What are you Hoarding in your Mental House?
- Prevent Dementia and Alzheimer's
- The Hundredth Monkey Cure – Cannabinoids
- Is There a Cure for Alcoholism?
- Color – The Hidden Persuader
- The Ultimate Healing – Integrative Memory and Past Lives Therapy®
- Take a Leap of Faith
- What I know for Sure
- ...and more

In the most delightful and warm way, Dr. Suka "talks" about the topics closest to our minds and hearts. This book includes transcripts from 24 of her recent Unity.FM international radio shows. You won't want to put this book down.

WORKBOOK (180 pages)
"Why Do I Feel This Way?" - **Natural Healing for Optimal Health and Relief from Moods and Depression** by Suka Chapel-Horst, RN, PhD, QMHP, CPLT

Moods, cravings, chronic depression, aches, pains and other symptoms are caused by treatable and reversible deficiencies in brain chemistry.

If your brain is low in "feel good" chemicals, you may experience moodiness, sadness, anxiety, overeating, insomnia, irritability, anger, lack of focus and concentration, poor memory, loneliness, decreased sex drive, lack of motivation, racing thoughts, suicidal thoughts, and more.

Find out which "feel good" brain chemicals you may be deficient in. Experience the power of amino acids to restore brain chemistry without medications. Discover the foods and basic food supplements that can restore your life to normal. The guidelines are clear, easy to understand and follow. This book may be all you need to achieve optimal health.

Avoid medication side effects, serious dangers, and addictive qualities. The only way to restore optimal health is by deleting poisonous nonfoods and feeding the brain the natural substances it needs to function normally.

The book includes:
- Ten Written Tests to Uncover the Underlying Cause
- Neurotransmitter Testing
- Amino Acid Formulas
- Nutritional Co-Factor Formulas
- Three Nutritional Programs
- Allergy and Candida Repair
- Seventeen Fun and Effective Stress-Reducing Exercises

WORKBOOK (180 pages)
How to Quit Drinking for Good and Feel Good
By Suka Chapel-Horst, RN, PhD, QMHP, CPLT

Live at Home

Keep it Private

Continue Normal Activities

Make it Affordable

Much of what we thought we knew about alcoholism and substance abuse is now obsolete. Advances in neuroscience, biochemistry, and psychology have found the underlying causes of all addictions and thirty-plus years of experience have given us the recovery method that is getting up to 85% recovery rates.

Shame, blame, and guilt be gone. Anger and hurt can change to healing, compassion and forgiveness when the real cause of addictions is understood. Addictions are not caused by a mental illness, nor are they caused by a lack of will power, a character defect, or a moral weakness.

Sobriety is not recovery. "One day at a time" struggling, white knuckling, dry drunk behaviors, depression, insomnia, anxiety, cravings, and other symptoms lead to relapse. With the new understanding of addictions, these, and other symptoms can be relieved and prevented, naturally, without the side effects and addictive qualities of prescription medications.

This book contains ten written tests to determine one's underlying biochemical imbalances and a step-by-step guide for gaining and maintaining lasting recovery without the symptoms that lead to relapse. Normal brain chemistry is restored with the natural building blocks of micronutrients and healthy nutrition. This program uses the most successful method of recovery available anywhere. Motivated and determined individuals can recover once and for all.

Written tests included in this book are:
- Alcohol Screening
- Carbohydrate Addiction
- Hypoglycemia
- Hypothyroid
- Candida
- Allergies
- Pyroluria
- High Histamine
- Low Histamine
- Attention Deficit (Hyperactivity) Disorder

These books and DVD's can be ordered through:
www.IMRIWellness.org
www.AriseAlcoholRecovery.com

DVD
Depression Cure
Ten Different Sources / Ten Different Approaches   Get Real Results
Your Guide to Finding and Treating the Real Underlying Cause
PowerPoint Presentation by Suka Chapel-Horst, RN, PhD, QMHP, CPLT

Don't waste time using the wrong approach to recovery. "Dr. Suka" pinpoints the different underlying sources of depression which must be treated uniquely and appropriately in order to fully recover without the use of pharmaceuticals. These inter-related causes require different treatment approaches to achieve permanent cure. Don't waste precious time, money, and hopes. Get to the root source from the start and find out how to recover naturally. DVD comes with a resource list.

BOTTOM LINE BOOKS

BOOK
Say Goodbye to Moods and Depression
A PowerPoint Presentation by Suka Chapel-Horst, RN, PhD, QMHP, CPLT

The only way to restore optimal health is by deleting poisonous nonfoods and feeding the brain the natural substances from which it is made.

Babies are made from food, not Prozac. After birth, why do we switch from the natural building blocks of life to synthetic pills? We can achieve optimal health when we remove the underlying brain chemical imbalances which lead to the symptoms of moods and depression including insomnia, anxiety, panic reactions, irritability, weight gain, aches and pains, and more.

The good news is that targeted micronutrients and healthy nutrition, along with other holistic methods of healthcare, can reduce or eliminate moods and depression, naturally.

BOOK
The Real Cause and Solution for Alcohol Addiction
The NEW Alcoholism Story
A PowerPoint Presentation by Suka Chapel-Horst, RN, PhD, QMHP, CPLT

Traditional thinking about alcohol addiction is now obsolete. Neuroscience, biochemistry, and psychology, plus over fifty-five years of experience, have given us a new and far more successful approach to recovery from this debilitating disorder.

The underlying *physical* cause of all addictions is either inherited or acquired imbalanced brain chemistry, and the underlying *psychological* cause of all addictions is unconscious, unresolved memories of traumatic experiences. Alcohol does not cause alcohol addiction. When the focus of addiction treatment is on the rebalancing of brain chemistry, plus belief management and memory therapy, recovery rates can soar.

BOOK/DVD
Wellness Simplified
How Food affects Moods, Bodies and Behaviors
A PowerPoint Presentation by Suka Chapel-Horst, RN, PhD, QMHP, CPLT

Think what you eat doesn't matter? Fast food, junk food, sodas, and pizza are the voices of violence, crime, and suicide, as well as obesity, joint pain, insomnia, anxiety, diabetes, depression, cancer, and *you name it!*

What we eat affects the quality of our lives. Sick and tired of feeling sick and tired? Are children's behaviors getting out of hand? Are school grades going down? It's OK. There's a solution and it's not rocket science.

This little book can change lives for the better, right now. The solution makes sense and it's doable. Say "goodbye" to moods, sickness, and unwanted behaviors. Say "hello" to good health and happiness.

BOOK

Cannabinoids – The Hundredth Monkey Cure
A PowerPoint Presentation by Suka Chapel-Horst, RN, PhD, QMHP, CPLT

The human body naturally produces cannabis-like chemicals that keep all body systems in balance. This internal cannabinoid system may be the most important health discovery of recent years. THC, CBN, and CBD from the cannabis sativa plant mimic our internal chemicals and work to improve our overall health. Cannabidiol, or CBD, cures or relieves symptoms of over 100 disorders. ...and it's legal everywhere because it doesn't have the psycho-active ingredient, THC.

Want better natural solutions for your health concerns? This DVD shows how to change brain chemistry and improve your life by using Cannabidiol (CBD), amino acids, neuro-nutrients, nutrition, exercise, and chronic stress reducers. Say goodbye to anxiety, stress, depression, insomnia, pain, physical disorders, and much more.

BOOK
The Gift – A Sound Mind for Life
A PowerPoint Presentation by Suka Chapel-Horst, RN, PhD, QMHP, CPLT

How to increase mental focus, improve memory, and prevent or delay Alzheimer's. Find out about the effects of stress and how to minimize it in order to prolong health and quality life. The DVD includes biochemical, nutritional, physical, emotional, and mental resources to minimize and delay the effects of aging. This is valuable information for any age.

BOOK
Trick or Treat – What Your Doctor isn't Telling You about Mood Altering Medications
A PowerPoint Presentation by Suka Chapel-Horst, RN, PhD, QMHP, CPLT

Is your doctor treating you or tricking you? If you are considering taking mood altering medications, are already on them, or want to get off them, you need to know what these medications are really doing to brain chemistry. Be informed in order to make wise decisions. Your emotional and mental life is at stake.

These books and DVD's can be ordered through:
www.IMRIWellness.org
www.AriseAlcoholRecovery.com

Suka Chapel-Horst

www.ingramcontent.com/pod-product-compliance
Lightning Source LLC
Chambersburg PA
CBHW070814290526

45795CB00002B/716